Freq

# all about
# carotenoids
## beta-carotene, lutein & lycopene

# JACK CHALLEM

## AVERY PUBLISHING GROUP
Garden City Park • New York

The information contained in this book is based upon the research and personal and professional experiences of the author. It is not intended as a substitute for consulting with your physician or other health care provider. Any attempt to diagnose and treat an illness should be done under the direction of a health care professional.

The publisher does not advocate the use of any particular health care protocol, but believes the information in this book should be available to the public. The publisher and author are not responsible for any adverse effects or consequences resulting from the use of any of the suggestions, preparations, or procedures discussed in this book. Should the reader have any questions concerning the appropriateness of any procedure or preparation mentioned, the author and the publisher strongly suggest consulting a professional health care advisor.

Series cover designer: Eric Macaluso
Cover image courtesy of Henkel Corporation

**Avery Publishing Group, Inc.**
120 Old Broadway, Garden City Park, NY 11040
1-800-548-5757 or visit us at www.averypublishing.com

ISBN: 0-89529-936-4

Printed in the United States of America

10   9   8   7   6   5   4   3   2

# Contents

# Introduction

In years past, mothers often advised their children to eat fruits and vegetables of many different colors, without knowing the reasons behind this advice. Today, scientists have provided an explanation of why "color" is good for health. Fruits and vegetables are rich in a family of plant pigments, called carotenoids, that have vitamin-like properties. Like vitamins, these colorful nutrients—which provide the orange, yellow, red, and other colors of fruits and vegetables—can promote good health and reduce the risk of disease.

You may have heard of some of these carotenoids, such as beta-carotene, lutein, and lycopene. Over the past twenty years, scientists and physicians have conducted hundreds of studies on these important nutrients. They have found, for example, that beta-carotene is a powerful stimulant of the immune cells that can protect against infections and cancer. Lutein may reduce the risk of macular degeneration, a leading cause of blindness among Americans over sixty-five. And lycopene may help prevent prostate cancer. These are just some of the many health benefits of carotenoids.

Why are carotenoids so beneficial to health? Carotenoids function as antioxidants, much like vitamins E and C. But we cannot live with just one or two antioxidants—our bodies seem to thrive when we consume many different antioxidants. And carotenoids are one of the largest groups of naturally occurring dietary antioxidants.

In *All About Carotenoids*, you'll learn about the principal carotenoids, as well as some of the minor ones, and their diverse roles in keeping you healthy. Recent scientific research will be explained in simple, understandable terms. You'll learn about the importance of eating a diet rich in carotenoids, and about the value of increasing your intake of specific carotenoid supplements. By the time you finish reading this book, you'll know that each of the individual carotenoids can provide health benefits—and that the sum of multiple, mixed carotenoids may provide even greater health benefits.

# 1.

# The Power of Carotenoids

Carotenoids are what make carrots orange, corn yellow, and tomatoes red. But in addition to making foods colorful and appealing, carotenoids have important health benefits that rival those of vitamins. In this chapter, you'll learn some of the basics about carotenoids. In subsequent chapters, you'll learn more about some of the important individual carotenoids.

## Q. What exactly is a carotenoid?

**A.** The term carotenoid (pronounced *cuh-rot-uh-noid*) refers to a family of about 600 different plant pigments. Despite the large number of carotenoids in nature, only a relatively small number of them play roles in human health. For example, around fifty carotenoids are found in the foods most Americans eat, but only fourteen have been identified in the bloodstream, an indicator of what is actually absorbed by the body. The other carotenoids are not absorbed, though it is still possible that they have some beneficial effects as they pass through the digestive tract. All carotenoids are fat-soluble nutrients, meaning that they can dissolve in fats and oils, but not water.

## Q. What's so special about carotenoids?

**A.** Many studies have found that an intake of high-carotenoid foods can reduce the risk of many different types of cancer, the second leading cause of death in the United States. Carotenoids may also lower the risk of heart disease, the number one cause of death. They have many other health benefits as well. Carotenoids can lower cholesterol levels and bolster resistance to sunburn. Increasing your intake of these nutrients can greatly reduce your risk of many diseases.

## Q. Are carotenoids essential nutrients?

**A.** Currently, carotenoids are not officially considered essential nutrients. However, there is substantial evidence that they are highly beneficial nutrients. Since the body cannot produce its own carotenoids, they have to be obtained from the diet.

People and other animals consumed large quantities of carotenoids over millions of years of evolution, and some researchers believe that people may have "coevolved" in a way that makes them dependent on carotenoids for good health.

Right now, it's hard to absolutely prove that carotenoids are essential. One reason is that researchers have tended to look for fairly rapid signs of nutritional deficiencies when carotenoid intake is decreased. However, heart disease and cancer take decades to develop, which makes it harder for scientists to connect a deficiency of a carotenoid with these disorders. With further study, many carotenoids may eventually be recognized as essential nutrients.

# Q. When were carotenoids discovered?

**A.** A scientist isolated "carotene" from the roots of carrots in 1831, and a few years later, another scientist identified "xanthophylls" in yellow autumn leaves. In 1911, yet another scientist recognized that these were related compounds, and he coined the term "carotenoids."

## Q. How did scientists discover the benefits of carotenoids?

**A.** Most nutrition researchers and health professionals recognize that diets rich in fruits and vegetables are associated with a relatively low risk of disease. For example, vegetarians have lower rates of heart disease and cancer compared with people who eat relatively few fruits and vegetables. And as we have learned, fruits and vegetables are rich sources of carotenoids, as well as many other important nutrients. Hundreds of studies have confirmed the general benefits of eating fruits and vegetables, and hundreds more have demonstrated how carotenoids contribute to health.

## Q. Does the body convert some carotenoids to vitamin A?

**A.** Yes, some dietary carotenoids are converted in your digestive tract to vitamin A, which is an essential nutrient—meaning that you cannot live without it. Beta-carotene is the best known carotenoid of this type and is sometimes referred to as provitamin A. Other major dietary carotenoids, such as lutein and lycopene, cannot be converted to vitamin A. In recent years, researchers have come to believe that the body does not convert carotenoids to vitamin A as efficiently as once thought.

## Q. Do I get enough carotenoids from my diet?

**A.** You would get enough dietary carotenoids if you ate at least five combined servings of fruits and vegetables each day. However, most Americans do not. The United States Department of Agriculture recommends that people consume three to five servings daily to reduce the risk of disease in general, and the National Cancer Institute recommends five to nine servings daily to reduce the risk of cancer. Still, the majority of Americans do not consume enough fruits and vegetables for optimum health.

Studies have found that only somewhere between 9 and 32 percent of Americans eat the recommended three to five daily servings of fruits and vegetables. Furthermore, most people who do eat fruits and vegetables eat from a very narrow group of these foods, so they lack a diverse selection of carotenoids. Ask yourself if you ate five combined servings of fruits and vegetables yesterday.

# Q. What role do carotenoids play in plants?

**A.** Carotenoids have a number of different functions in plants. Sunlight is necessary for plants to grow. However, ultraviolet (UV) wavelengths can generate dangerous molecules called free radicals, which injure living cells. Free radicals oxidize cells much the way they turn iron to rust or turn butter rancid. Carotenoids function as antioxidants, which means they protect against free radicals. So, in other words, carotenoids are a plant's defense against free radicals. Carotenoids also influence the behavior of plant genes, which direct the behavior of cells.

# Q. What happens when we eat carotenoids?

**A.** When we eat carotenoids, we acquire the same antioxidant benefits that plants do from these substances. Similar to essential nutrients, carotenoids play many other roles in health as well, such as enhancing your resistance to infection; preventing damage to your deoxyribonucleic acid (DNA), or genetic material; and reducing your risk of cancer.

## Q. Then why don't people eat more fruits and vegetables?

**A.** This is an admirable goal, but it is very difficult to change people's eating habits. Some people just don't like the taste of vegetables such as broccoli and spinach. Indeed, researchers have discovered that large numbers of people are "supertasters"— people who are more sensitive to bitter tastes—and so avoid eating vegetables. Other people find it more convenient to eat a hamburger and fries than to eat fruits and vegetables. (While made from potatoes, fries are high in oxidized fats.) Still other people never developed the habit of eating fresh fruits and vegetables.

## Q. Can supplements compensate for a diet lacking in fruits and vegetables?

**A.** Various types of carotenoid supplements can partly make up for such a diet. Of course, no supplement can provide all of the beneficial nutrients found in foods. But studies have found that carotenoid supplements can reduce the risk of disease in people who do not usually eat fruits and vegetables.

High doses of some carotenoid supplements in addition to a regular diet of fruits and vegetables may also reduce the risk of some diseases. For example, beta-carotene supplements can reverse a precancerous condition called oral leukoplakia, lutein supplements may reduce the risk and perhaps slow the progression of macular degeneration, and lycopene supplements can reduce the risk of prostate cancer.

## Q. Aren't carotenoids better absorbed from foods than from supplements?

**A.** Actually, it's just the opposite: carotenoids in supplement form are better absorbed than carotenoids from foods. The reason is that carotenoids in foods are locked in a fibrous matrix that is difficult for the body to break down. Cooking foods helps break down this matrix, increasing carotenoid absorption—though overcooking can break down the carotenoids themselves. Because carotenoids in dietary supplements do not contain this matrix, they are very well absorbed. Several scientific studies have demonstrated this to be true.

# Q. What kinds of carotenoid supplements are available?

**A.** There are several major types. Beta-carotene is found in both natural and synthetic forms. The source of natural beta-carotene is typically a type of algae, such as *Dunaliella salina*, and this is usually identified on the label. Natural lutein and lycopene are also found in dietary supplements. There are also "mixed" carotenoids, which contain an assortment of natural carotenoids, usually from algae or palm oil. In the following chapters, I'll discuss these major dietary carotenoids in more detail.

# 2.

# Beta-Carotene

Beta-carotene is one of the most common carotenoids found in foods and is the primary precursor to vitamin A, meaning that the body can convert it to vitamin A. Its orange-like color accounts for the appearance of some fruits and vegetables, such as carrots, pumpkins, peaches, and sweet potatoes. Studies have shown that beta-carotene can have diverse and sometimes surprising health benefits. For example, it can strengthen the immune system, provide protection against some types of cancer, and reduce the risk of sun damage.

## Q. When did researchers first realize that beta-carotene has health benefits?

**A.** For decades, scientists have recognized that beta-carotene can be converted by the body to vitamin A, and therefore can provide the same health benefits supplied by that essential nutrient. For instance, both vitamin A and beta-carotene can be used to treat night blindness, an early sign of vitamin-A deficiency in which the eyes do not quickly adjust to changes in light. However, it has been found that beta-carotene works more slowly to correct this condition because the body must first convert it to vitamin A.

During the 1970s, researchers accumulated considerable evidence that fruits and vegetables rich in beta-carotene can reduce the risk of heart disease and some types of cancer. Their research also revealed that many of beta-carotene's health benefits are independent of its vitamin A effects.

## Q. What are the benefits of taking beta-carotene supplements?

A. Beta-carotene supplements provide a number of key health benefits. Perhaps beta-carotene's most significant benefit is its ability to activate some of the body's immune cells. Beta-carotene also increases lung capacity, meaning that it enables you to breathe in and exhale more air—signs of good respiratory health. There's also evidence that beta-carotene can reduce DNA damage, provide protection from the sun, and lessen the risk of some types of cancer. It also can lower cholesterol levels and may lower the risk of heart disease. Beta-carotene is also a safe source of vitamin A—which can be toxic in high doses—because the body converts beta-carotene to vitamin A slowly.

## Q. How do beta-carotene supplements improve immune function?

**A.** Beta-carotene improves immune function in a number of different ways. In one recent study, David A. Hughes, PhD, and his colleagues at the Institute of Food Research, England, studied how beta-carotene influenced the effectiveness of mono-cytes—one type of immune cell that seeks out and helps destroy cancer cells and infectious microbes.

In order to distinguish a cancer cell from normal cells, monocytes have to be able to tell them apart. The monocyte's cancer detector is a protein called MHC II, which sits on the surface of the cell. In a sense, it's a form of anticancer radar. When the MHC II protein detects a cancer cell, the monocyte sends a signal to other immune cells, which move in and destroy the abnormal cells. However, if mono-cytes don't have enough MHC II proteins, the cancer cells go by unnoticed and can then replicate more cancer cells.

This is where beta-carotene comes in. According to a study by Dr. Hughes, beta-carotene increases the number of MHC II proteins on monocytes. He discovered this in a study of twenty-five healthy men who were given either beta-carotene supplements or a placebo—an inactive look-alike supplement—for thirty days. Men taking 15 mg of beta-carotene daily developed large numbers of cancer-detecting MHC II proteins on their monocytes.

## Q. Did beta-carotene supplements help these men in any other way?

**A.** Yes, they did. Dr. Hughes found that beta-carotene supplements also increased the men's production of tumor necrosis factor alpha (TNF-a), an immune-system molecule that, like a heat-seeking missile, zeroes in on cancer cells and destroys them.

## Q. How else do beta-carotene supplements enhance the immune system?

**A.** A number of studies at Tufts University, Medford, Massachusetts, have found that beta-carotene supplements increase the activity of natural killer (NK) cells. NK cells are powerful immune cells that attack both cancer cells and virus-infected cells. The Tufts researchers have found that beta-carotene supplements boost NK cell activity, particularly in elderly men. This is important because immune function declines with age. In one recent study, elderly men who had taken 50 mg of beta-carotene every other day for twelve years had significantly greater NK cell activity.

Researchers at Loyola University Medical Center in Maywood, Illinois, recently found that beta-carotene supplements (30 mg daily) increased immune function in fifty patients with colon cancers or colon polyps. Before taking beta-carotene, the colon cancer patients had lower percentages of CD4, interleukin-2 (IL-2), and interleukin-2 positive (IL-2R) immune cells. These cells play important roles in preventing and fighting cancer. Beta-carotene supplements significantly increased the number of IL-2R and CD4 cells in the colon cancer patients and slightly increased IL-2R and CD4 cells in patients with polyps. Larger numbers of these cells may enhance the body's ability to destroy cancer cells.

## Q. Can beta-carotene supplements keep me from getting easily sunburned?

**A.** There's a good chance that they can. In a

German study, researchers asked twenty young women to take either 30 mg of beta-carotene or a placebo daily for ten weeks. They were then asked, under scientifically controlled situations, to sunbathe at various times over a thirteen-day period. While sunbathing, the women used a topical sunscreen cream. The women who had taken beta-carotene supplements and used sunscreen had less sunburn than those using a topical sunscreen alone.

## Q. How do beta-carotene supplements help protect me from the sun's harmful rays?

**A.** Ultraviolet rays in sunlight generate large numbers of free radicals, which damage skin cells. The skin is rich in a number of antioxidants, including beta-carotene, vitamin E, and vitamin C. These antioxidants are quickly used up neutralizing free radicals. Supplements of beta-carotene bolster the antioxidants in the skin, so the skin is better able to withstand and counteract free radicals. A very recent study found that women who took natural beta-carotene had significant increases in beta-carotene stores in skin throughout the body.

# Q. Can beta-carotene protect me from skin cancer?

**A.** Beta-carotene supplements may reduce the long-term risk of skin cancer, though there are no studies that have yet proved this. We do know that excessive exposure to sunlight increases the risk of skin cancer and that skin cancer probably begins with free-radical damage. By reducing free-radical damage, beta-carotene should reduce the risk of skin cancer.

In addition, excessive exposure to sunlight suppresses the body's immune system, which limits its ability to protect against cancer cells. Again, beta-carotene supplements seem to prevent sunlight-induced immune suppression.

Skin damage from sunlight begins to take place within a couple minutes of exposure, so it is best to limit your exposure to sunlight to fifteen minutes or less daily—after all, a little sunlight is good for health. But if you spend a lot of time outdoors in the sun, it would be prudent to take supplements of beta-carotene and perhaps other antioxidants, such as vitamins C and E. Of course, it's also smart to cover your skin to minimize skin damage from sunlight and to use sunscreen on all exposed areas.

## Q. Can beta-carotene supplements protect me against any other type of cancer?

**A.** There is considerable evidence that beta-carotene does provide protection against many other types of cancer. For example, there is evidence based on a number of human studies conducted at the University of Arizona, Tucson, and other research centers that beta-carotene can help reverse a condition called oral leukoplakia, a precancerous lesion of the mouth or throat that often leads to full-blown oral cancer if left untreated. Vitamin A and vitamin E can also reverse oral leukoplakia, which occurs most often in people who smoke tobacco and drink excessive amounts of alcohol.

## Q. How does beta-carotene help prevent cancer?

**A.** As an antioxidant, beta-carotene quenches singlet oxygen and other types of free radicals. In doing so, it prevents free radicals from damaging your cells' DNA. Damaged DNA incorrectly replicates genetic instructions, accelerating the aging of cells and increasing the risk of various diseases. For instance, it is damaged DNA that creates cancer cells and instructs them to grow uncontrollably.

In one study, Japanese researchers took human lymphocyte cells from healthy young women and then exposed the cells to x-ray radiation. Radiation creates free radicals and increases cell damage, essentially speeding up a natural process of cell damage that occurs with age. However, when the women took beta-carotene supplements, their cells became more resistant to x-ray damage. Other experiments have shown similar benefits. For example, researchers have also found that cells are better able to recover from DNA damage if they have been saturated with beta-carotene.

Keep in mind that beta-carotene plays a role in preventing some cancers, but not others—and that there is no evidence to indicate that it can help treat active cancers.

## Q. Can beta-carotene help reduce the risk of breast cancer?

**A.** There is strong evidence that diets high in fresh fruits and vegetables can reduce the risk of most cancers, including breast cancer. Scientists have tried to gauge the relative importance of different nutrients in fruits and vegetables, and have found that beta-carotene and other carotenoids are associated with a reduced risk of developing breast cancer.

In one recent study, researchers at Harvard University and Tufts University studied 109 Boston-area women who had breast biopsies. The researchers found that women with higher breast concentrations of carotenoids were less likely to have breast cancer. In contrast, women with breast cancer had significantly lower levels of beta-carotene, lycopene, lutein, and zeaxanthin in their breast tissue. Women with the highest breast levels of beta-carotene had the lowest risk of breast cancer. Keep in mind, though, that this study showed an association, not a cause and effect.

Other studies have shown similar trends. For example, researchers have found that women who ate carrots or spinach more than twice weekly had a 44-percent lower risk of developing breast cancer, compared with women who did not consume any of these vegetables. Women with the highest intake of beta-carotene in foods had a 36-percent lower risk of breast cancer.

## Q. Can beta-carotene also provide protection against cervical dysplasia and cancer of the cervix?

**A.** Several studies have found that beta-carotene may lower the risk of these conditions. Cervical dysplasia is a precancerous condition in which large numbers of cervical cells are abnormal but not actually cancerous. In a study at the University of Arizona Cancer Center, Tucson, researchers found that out of ten nutrients analyzed, only low beta-carotene levels appeared to be associated with cervical dysplasia and cancer of the cervix.

In a laboratory study, Japanese researchers found that the natural form of beta-carotene was more effective than the synthetic form of beta-carotene in stopping the growth of cervical dysplasia cells. This study is one of many that point to a clear difference in the effects of natural and synthetic beta-carotene. I'll discuss these differences in more detail further on in this chapter.

## Q. Can beta-carotene help prevent prostate cancer?

**A.** Two carotenoids, beta-carotene and lycopene, seem to reduce the risk of prostate cancer. (I'll discuss lycopene in Chapter 4.) In an ongoing study of male physicians, Meir Stampfer, MD, of Harvard Medical School assessed the effects of diets high in beta-carotene, diets low in beta-carotene, and diets that included beta-carotene supplements (50 mg every other day) over twelve years in several thousand male doctors.

Men who had low blood levels of beta-carotene because they ate few fruits and vegetables were one-third more likely to develop prostate cancer. However, if the men not eating fruits and vegetables took beta-carotene supplements, they had a 36-percent lower-than-average risk of prostate cancer. In other words, the beta-carotene supplements made up for the lack of fruits and vegetables in the diet, at least in terms of prostate health.

## Q. Is beta-carotene of value in other types of cancer?

**A.** Beta-carotene seems to be beneficial in reducing the risk of other types of cancer as well as those mentioned previously. There is promising animal and cell-culture research suggesting that beta-carotene can reduce the risk of colon cancer, liver cancer, and pancreatic cancer.

Beta-carotene supplements taken with other antioxidants may have an even greater role in cancer prevention. In one study, researchers gave a combination of beta-carotene, vitamin E, and selenium to more than 3,000 people with esophageal dysplasia, a precancerous condition. The supplement combination reduced the risk of both esophageal cancer and cancer-related death.

## Q. What is the controversy surrounding beta-carotene and lung cancer?

**A.** In 1994, Finnish researchers reported the results of the Alpha-Tocopherol Beta-Carotene Cancer Prevention Study Group (ATBC), which found that beta-carotene supplementation slightly increased the risk of lung cancer in men who were smokers or asbestos workers. And in 1996, American researchers announced the results of the Beta-Carotene and Retinol Efficacy Trial (CARET), which found that high supplemental doses of beta-carotene and vitamin A increased the risk of lung cancer in smokers.

These findings surprised many people because they contradicted what was generally believed— that beta-carotene would reduce the risk of cancer. While the results of these studies have not been shown to be inaccurate, medical research can sometimes be distorted, incompletely reported to the public, or contradicted by further studies.

# Q. What other information would shed more light on these findings?

A. The findings of the CARET and ATBC studies were not as conclusive as some media reports would have the public believe.

The CARET study research also revealed that former smokers who took 30 mg of beta-carotene and 25,000 IU of vitamin A daily were 20-percent less likely to develop lung cancer. It further revealed that men with the highest blood levels of beta-carotene at the start of the study were 40-percent less likely to develop lung cancer. However, these positive findings were downplayed by the researchers.

Upon further analysis of the data, the Finnish researchers involved in the ATBC study found that a combination of beta-carotene, smoking, and high alcohol consumption increased the risk of lung cancer by 35 percent. However, beta-carotene did *not* increase the risk of lung cancer among people who smoked less than a pack of cigarettes daily or drank little or no alcohol. In other words, beta-carotene was not harmful as long as the men did not smoke or drink excessively.

This later finding was consistent with that of a study of American physicians, which found that beta-carotene supplements had no effect, good or bad, on lung cancer. This same study found a decrease in the risk of prostate cancer, indicating that a nutrient that protects against one type of cancer may not protect against a different type of cancer.

In the CARET study, men who smoked and consumed three or more alcoholic drinks daily had twice the risk of lung cancer if they also took very high daily doses of beta-carotene, plus very high daily doses of vitamin A for many years. High doses of vitamin A can be toxic, and combined with beta-carotene's ability to convert to vitamin A, the subjects may have been taking the equivalent of 60,000 IU of vitamin A—an extremely high dose that can lead to vitamin A toxicity within a few weeks.

## Q. What are the most important points to remember about these two studies?

**A.** It is important to remember that people who smoked and drank a relatively small amount had no increase in lung cancer risk when taking beta-carotene supplements in the ATBC study. Only people who were smoking and drinking in excess—really abusing their bodies—had problems with beta-carotene supplementation, and most probably would have had serious health problems even if they had not taken beta-carotene. Also keep in mind that former smokers had a substantial reduction in lung cancer risk when they took beta-carotene supplements.

Both smoking and alcohol can overwhelm the body's antioxidants—in effect, they oxidize the antioxidants. The oxidized byproducts of beta-carotene—that is, the compounds created when alcohol damages beta-carotene—increase the liver toxicity of alcohol. Similarly, cigarette smoke contains large numbers of free radicals, which also appear to damage beta-carotene. In other words, beta-carotene is no match for people who are heavy smokers and hard drinkers.

There is strong evidence, however, that when beta-carotene is consumed in combination with other antioxidants, such as vitamin E and selenium, the nutrients form a stronger antioxidant network that helps the body resist free-radical damage. Perhaps the researchers of the two studies on lung cancer and beta-carotene supplementation had hoped that beta-carotene would be a silver bullet cure for lung cancer. The reality is that nutrients, in contrast to drugs, work best as a team.

# Q. Did these studies use natural or synthetic beta-carotene?

**A.** These two studies used synthetic beta-carotene. This is a very important point because the synthetic form of beta-carotene does not have the same antioxidant properties of natural beta-carotene. Some researchers believe that the results of these studies would have been much more positive if natural beta-carotene, or a mix of carotenoids, had been used instead of the synthetic form. The difference between the natural and synthetic forms will be discussed in more detail further on in this chapter.

## Q. Do beta-carotene supplements have any positive effects on lung function?

**A.** A researcher, John R. Balmes, MD, of the University of California, San Francisco, analyzed a subgroup of 816 men in the CARET study. He found that beta-carotene had a positive effect on lung capacity—even among smokers and men exposed to asbestos dust. Typically, such people have poor lung function, but beta-carotene and vitamin A supplements improved their lung function contrary to the CARET and ATBC studies.

Several other studies have found that beta-carotene supplements, sometimes combined with other antioxidants, improve lung function. In one study, Patricia Cassano, PhD, of Cornell University found that beta-carotene stood out among other nutrients for its association with normal lung function. In another study, researchers found that a combination of beta-carotene, vitamin C, and vitamin E improved several indicators of lung function in people working outdoors in Mexico City, one of the world's most polluted cities.

## Q. Since beta-carotene seems to have some positive effects on lung function, would it also help relieve symptoms of asthma?

**A.** Beta-carotene supplements may also benefit people with asthma. Asthmatics suffer from oxidative stress—they have relatively high levels of free radicals in their bodies compared with the levels of antioxidants. A number of studies have found that antioxidants such as vitamin C are helpful in reducing asthmatic symptoms, but the research relating to beta-carotene's antioxidant effects on asthma is still preliminary. In a promising Israeli study, thirty-eight patients with exercise-induced asthma took either beta-carotene supplements or a placebo. Asthmatic patients taking the placebo developed breathing problems after exercising, but more than half of the asthmatic patients taking beta-carotene were protected against exercise-induced asthma.

## Q. Why does it seem that some studies on beta-carotene's effect on lung function contradict others?

**A.** Contradiction is sometimes the nature of scientific research. But there are two important things to remember about beta-carotene. The first important point is that beta-carotene supplements, as well as vitamins and minerals, can do wonders for health—but they can't magically restore an abused body to good health. So, if you smoke and drink, either stop or cut down. The second point is that there may be an ideal dosage of beta-carotene for heavy smokers and excessive drinkers, but further studies are needed.

## Q. Can beta-carotene help reduce the risk of heart disease?

**A.** Although the scientific evidence is sometimes contradictory—this, again, is often the nature of scientific research—there is compelling research that beta-carotene can lower cholesterol levels and thereby reduce the risk of heart disease. Beta-carotene's benefits to the heart seem to increase when it is combined with other antioxidant nutrients.

A recent study by Stephen B. Kritchevsky, PhD, published in the *American Journal of Clinical Nutrition*, found that diets high in beta-carotene could reduce the risk of heart disease by about one-third in female smokers. Another study, by George W. Comstock, MD, found that beta-carotene stood out among other carotenoids for its association with a low risk of heart disease.

## Q. How does beta-carotene affect cholesterol?

A. First, remember that cholesterol is essential for life. It is the basic building block of some of your body's steroid hormones. Your body also uses cholesterol to make vitamin D. While very high cholesterol levels might indicate a problem, it is the oxidative damage—caused by too many free radicals or not enough antioxidants—to the low-density lipoprotein (LDL) form of cholesterol that seems to play a key role in the development of heart disease.

White blood cells seem to sense that oxidized LDL is harmful to the body, so they attack and consume it as they would invading bacteria. But these

LDL-engorged white blood cells can get stuck to the walls of the artery, where they start forming cholesterol deposits. Therefore one of the important steps in preventing heart disease is to prevent the oxidation of LDL, which can be done by taking beta-carotene supplements and other antioxidants. In a study published in the *American Journal of Clinical Nutrition*, researchers calculated that, at least in women, 5.37 mg (8,950 IU) of beta-carotene could protect against LDL oxidation.

Also, researchers at the University of Toronto found that 20 mg of beta-carotene daily reduced lipid peroxidation in smokers. Lipid peroxidation is the term for oxidized, or free-radical-damaged, fats, which are higher in those people who are at risk for heart disease. Another study, conducted at the University of Washington, Seattle, found that supplements of beta-carotene, vitamin E, and vitamin C in tomato juice reduce LDL oxidation in smokers.

There is also intriguing animal research that suggests that beta-carotene can lower cholesterol levels. Judy A. Driskell, PhD, of the University of Nebraska, Lincoln, fed rabbits—common laboratory models for studying heart disease—a diet that promotes heart disease. She also supplemented the rabbits' diet with beta-carotene, vitamin E, or a combination of the two.

Beta-carotene and vitamin E seemed to have complementary effects. Beta-carotene decreased total cholesterol levels and LDL levels, the size of cholesterol deposits, and the thickness of blood vessel walls. While beta-carotene did not actually reduce LDL oxidation in this study, vitamin E did.

## Q. What exactly is night blindness, and how can beta-carotene help?

**A.** Night blindness is a fairly common condition indicating vitamin-A deficiency in which the eyes do not quickly adjust to changes in light. For example, people with night blindness have difficulty seeing when they walk from daylight into a dark movie theater, and must wait several minutes for their eyes to adjust. Similarly, the glare of oncoming headlights can blind nighttime drivers who have night blindness.

Night blindness may precede some very serious eye diseases that can lead to complete blindness. Among these diseases are glaucoma and retinitis pigmentosa.

Because of beta-carotene's ability to be slowly converted to vitamin A in the body, it can have the same beneficial effects of vitamin A in reversing this condition, though it may take longer.

# Q. Does beta-carotene provide any other health benefits?

**A.** Yes. A study conducted at Johns Hopkins University, Baltimore, examined the blood levels of antioxidants in patients and years later compared them with the long-term health of the subjects. The researchers found that blood levels of beta-carotene, vitamin C, and vitamin A were consistently lower in patients who were later diagnosed with rheumatoid arthritis and lupus erythematosus—both autoimmune disorders. Beta-carotene levels, especially, of those with rheumatoid arthritis showed a statistically significant difference. On average, people who developed rheumatoid arthritis originally had 29-percent lower blood levels of beta-carotene than those subjects who remained in good health. This doesn't mean that beta-carotene is a treatment for rheumatoid arthritis. It does, however, show that inadequate intake over many years may increase the risk of this disease and possibly others.

# Q. What's the difference between natural and synthetic beta-carotene?

**A.** Natural beta-carotene consists of two molecules

called isomers. One isomer is 9-cis beta-carotene, and the other isomer is all-trans beta-carotene. These isomers contain the same molecules, but the molecules are arranged differently—kind of like the different shapes of snowflakes. Isomers commonly have very different chemical and biological properties. For example, the B vitamin inositol and glucose are isomers of each other, but they perform very different functions in the body.

According to Ami Ben-Amotz, PhD, a beta-carotene researcher at Israel's National Institute of Oceanography, the 9-cis form of beta-carotene is the primary antioxidant part of the molecule. But synthetic beta-carotene does not contain the 9-cis forms of beta-carotene. It consists only of the all-trans form of beta-carotene, which is a very weak antioxidant.

## Q. How common is the 9-cis form of beta-carotene in foods?

**A.** A recent study by Dr. Ben-Amotz found that the 9-cis form of beta-carotene formed a substantial portion of the total beta-carotene in lettuce, parsley, sweet potatoes, and many other foods. But the 9-cis form of beta-carotene is only one of the myriad forms of beta-carotene and other carotenoids found in foods.

# Q. Why don't we hear more about the 9-cis form of beta-carotene?

**A.** Blood measurements are probably the most common way of analyzing nutrient absorption in the blood, but researchers have had difficulty measuring the 9-cis form of beta-carotene using this procedure. Some of the 9-cis in the blood seems to convert quickly to other forms of beta-carotene, and some of the 9-cis appears to be absorbed into tissues so rapidly that it cannot be easily measured with today's technology. It does, however, show up in other parts of the body, such as in breast milk. One researcher believes that the presence of 9-cis in breast milk may indicate that it has a very important, but little studied, biological role.

# Q. What should I look for when buying natural beta-carotene supplements?

**A.** You should read the labels on the bottles of beta-carotene supplements, mixed carotenoid supplements, antioxidant formulas, and multivitamins for their beta-carotene content. The richest natural supplemental sources are generally algae, which might be identified on the label as *Dunaliella salina*, as *D. salina,* or as some related type of algae. These types of algae are grown to be rich sources of beta-carotene. They naturally contain 40 to 50 percent of the desirable 9-cis form of beta-carotene, around 50 percent of the natural all-trans form of beta-carotene, and small amounts of other carotenoids, including alpha-carotene, lutein, zeaxanthin, and cryptoxanthin.

# Q. What's the best way to take beta-carotene supplements?

**A.** Carotenoids seem to work best together, so it is probably better to take a mix of carotenoids that includes beta-carotene. After all, a mix more closely resembles what you would consume in a diet that includes fruits and vegetables. Mixed carotenoids will be discussed in Chapter 6.

Carotenoids also seem to work well with other antioxidants, so the best situation might be to take beta-carotene supplements as part of a mixed carotenoid supplement and as part of a multi-antioxidant formula. Of course, it would be better yet to take all dietary supplements in conjunction with a diet rich in fruits and vegetables.

# Q. What's the ideal dosage of beta-carotene?

**A.** The ideal dosage of beta-carotene for most adults should be about 15 mg daily. Some supplement labels may list beta-carotene in terms of international units, and in that case, the ideal dosage would be 25,000 IU. I'll explain more about these measurements in Chapter 6.

# 3.

# Lutein and Zeaxanthin

Lutein (pronounced *loo-teen*) rivals beta-caro-tene as one of the most common carotenoids found in the American diet. It provides the rich yellow color of corn and egg yolks. Lutein is also found in kale, spinach, and broccoli, but darker pigments also contained in these foods mask its yellow color. Recent studies have found that lutein is virtually essential for normal vision, and may play an important role in the prevention of heart disease and in the reduction of breast cancer. Zeaxanthin (pronounced *zee-uh-zan-thin*), which is found in okra, cress leaf, and chicory leaf, is closely related to lutein and shares its beneficial effects. In addition to getting zeaxanthin from some foods, the body can convert some lutein to zeaxanthin.

# Q. What kind of carotenoids are lutein and zeaxanthin?

**A.** Lutein and zeaxanthin have slightly different chemical structures than beta-carotene, and are technically known as xanthophylls—a subgroup of carotenoids. Both of these nutrients are commonly found in the American diet. Depending on the types of fruits and vegetables in your diet, you may actually consume more lutein than beta-carotene. Like beta-carotene, lutein is a fat-soluble, antioxidant nutrient.

# Q. Is lutein considered an essential nutrient?

**A.** While lutein is not currently recognized as an essential nutrient, this may change within the next few years. The majority of studies involving lutein have focused on its effect upon the eyes, and the results suggest that lutein is required for normal vision.

# Q. How are lutein and zeaxanthin involved in eye health?

**A.** Light passes through the lens of your eye and is focused on the back of your eye—an area known as the retina. The retina is somewhat like a movie screen onto which images are projected. The retina changes these light images into electrical impulses that are then transmitted to the brain by the optic nerve.

At the center of the retina is a small area known as the macula, which is the part of the eye responsible for detailed vision. The macula contains a pigment known as the macular pigment, which consists primarily of lutein and zeaxanthin—the only carotenoids to be identified in the macular pigment. This suggests that these nutrients play an important role in eye health.

## Q. What does the macular pigment do?

**A.** In addition to picking up fine detail, the yellowish macular pigment filters out harmful wavelengths of blue light, which can generate damaging free radicals in the eye. As antioxidants, the lutein and zeaxanthin in the macular pigment also seem to reduce the amount of damage caused by free-radical damage in this part of the eye.

# Q. What is macular degeneration, and how does it develop in the eye?

**A.** Macular degeneration—the leading cause of blindness among Americans over age sixty-five—is the deterioration of the macula, the part of the eye responsible for central vision. The macular pigment becomes too thin to filter out all of the harmful blue wavelengths, and at the same time, there is an increase in drusen—an oxidized fat—in the eye. Both a thin macular pigment and an increase in drusen are indicative of macular degeneration. People with macular degeneration tend to have thin macular pigments and low lutein blood levels, probably resulting from low lutein intakes.

Macular degeneration causes complete blindness in 300,000 Americans and a partial loss of vision in an estimated 13 million others per year.

# Q. Can lutein help treat macular degeneration?

**A.** Many studies strongly suggest that lutein can help treat macular degeneration, but so far, no human studies have clearly demonstrated this. It is probably not possible to reverse advanced macular degeneration, but researchers believe that a high intake of lutein supplements or lutein-rich foods will slow the progression of this disease. It is conceivable that large amounts of lutein may reverse the early stages of macular degeneration.

There have been a number of studies showing that eating high-lutein diets or taking 30 mg daily of lutein supplements can significantly increase the thickness of the macular pigment within about five months. In one study, the macular pigment increased by as much as 39 percent. This increase would decrease the amount of harmful blue wavelengths by 40 percent.

In another study, described in the *Journal of the American Medical Association*, researchers found that people consuming the largest quantity of lutein-rich vegetables—about 6 mg of lutein daily—have the lowest risk of macular degeneration.

# Q. Isn't the thickness of the macular pigment related to genetics?

**A.** Genetics plays an important role in all disease risks, including macular degeneration. However, in a study of identical twins, researchers found that the thickness of the macular pigment varied from individual to individual, most likely because of different eating habits.

## Q. Can lutein help prevent cataracts and other eye problems?

**A.** Lutein, which is the only carotenoid that has been identified in the lens of the eye, may help to prevent the formation of a cataract—the clouding of the lens. The inside of the eye is bathed in a rich solution of antioxidants, including lutein, glutathione, vitamin C, and vitamin E. These antioxidants protect the eye from damaging ultraviolet radiation. People who don't consume enough fruits and vegetables containing these antioxidants lack optimal levels of eye protection and, therefore, have a higher risk of developing eye disorders.

## Q. Does lutein have any cardiovascular benefits?

**A.** As an antioxidant, lutein reduces the oxidation of LDL cholesterol (the "bad" cholesterol), which in turn should reduce the risk of heart disease and other cardiovascular diseases. In comparing the diets of people living in Toulouse, France, with those of people living in Belfast, Ireland, researchers noted that the relatively low risk of heart disease in Toulouse was linked to high blood levels of lutein and cryptoxanthin, another carotenoid. In contrast, low levels of these carotenoids were associated with a higher risk of heart disease in Belfast.

## Q. Does lutein offer any benefits in breast cancer reduction?

**A.** Studies suggest that lutein may offer some protection against breast cancer. In experiments at Washington State University, Boon P. Chew, PhD, fed laboratory mice a diet with different amounts of supplemental lutein or a diet completely lacking in lutein. After two weeks, all of the mice were injected with breast cancer cells. Those mice that received lutein as part of their diet developed breast cancer later than did untreated animals. The lutein-fed mice also had a lower incidence of breast tumors, and had tumors of lesser size than those of untreated mice.

## Q. How much supplemental lutein should I take?

**A.** For general health maintenance, 4 to 6 mg of lutein daily should be sufficient. However, if you are trying to enhance your protection against macular degeneration, 30 to 40 mg of lutein daily might be helpful. Because lutein is a fat-soluble nutrient, and fat enhances the absorption of lutein, be sure to eat it with small amounts of oily or fatty food. If your body cannot take fats and oils, take lutein with your regular meal.

## Q. Should I also take supplemental zeaxanthin for eye health?

**A.** Zeaxanthin is not available alone in supplemental form. Since the body can convert some of its lutein to zeaxanthin, and lutein supplements generally contain zeaxanthin, it is not necessary to take additional zeaxanthin. But the most sensible approach to protect eye health is to eat a diet containing a lot of carotenoid-rich foods. And, if you are at risk of macular degeneration, it might be worthwhile to also take lutein supplements, which should also provide zeaxanthin.

## Q. Are lutein supplements available over the counter?

**A.** Like beta-carotene supplements, lutein is available over the counter and without a prescription in pharmacies and health food stores. It is, after all, a natural component of many foods. There is some natural zeaxanthin in these supplements, as well.

## Q. What kind of lutein supplements are available?

**A.** Two types of lutein supplements are available on the market; both are derived from marigold petals—a rich, natural source of lutein. In fact, some of these lutein products are marketed as marigold extracts. One type of lutein consists of free lutein—pure, crystalline lutein. The other type is lutein ester, which occurs naturally in many common foods. (An ester is a type of compound that adds chemical stability—and lengthens the shelf life—of natural products.) Both free lutein and lutein ester are absorbed very well by the body. However, there is some preliminary evidence, based on research conducted at the University of Illinois, that lutein ester may be assimilated and retained by the body a little better than free lutein.

# 4.

# Lycopene

---

Lycopene (pronounced *like-o-peen*), another common carotenoid, gives foods such as tomatoes their red color. In fact, tomatoes are the richest dietary source of lycopene. And, as strange as it may sound, eating tomato sauce has been associated with a lower risk of prostate cancer, and may even reduce the risk of other types of cancer and heart disease. Smaller amounts of lycopene are found in watermelon, pink grapefruit, guava, and apricots.

## Q. What's the big news about lycopene?

**A.** Lycopene grabbed headlines a few years ago when researchers reported that diets high in this carotenoid significantly reduced the risk of prostate cancer. Edward Giovannucci, MD, of Harvard Medical School, analyzed the dietary habits of almost

48,000 male physicians and their risk of prostate cancer. Giovannucci found that four foods were associated with a low risk of developing prostate cancer. These foods were tomato sauce on spaghetti, pizza with tomato sauce, uncooked tomatoes, and strawberries.

Men who consumed some form of tomato other than tomato juice two or more times per week were 21- to 34-percent less likely to develop prostate cancer than men who ate very few or no tomato products at all. Men who ate more than ten servings of tomato products weekly had a 45-percent lower risk of developing prostate cancer.

## Q. Why did some forms of tomato prove to be more beneficial than others in this study?

A. The greatest benefits derived from tomatoes were associated with spaghetti sauce and pizza sauce, followed by uncooked tomatoes. There are a couple of reasons for this, which have been confirmed by subsequent research.

One reason why tomato sauces were associated with the greatest health benefits is that they actually contain more digestible lycopene than uncooked tomatoes. Lycopene is normally locked into the fibrous matrix of uncooked tomatoes, which is difficult for the body to break down during digestion. The heat of cooking helps break down this matrix, thereby releasing more bioavailable lycopene.

Another reason is that lycopene is a fat-soluble nutrient, requiring some dietary fat or oil for absorption. Typically, tomato sauces are made with olive oil, which makes absorption of lycopene possible. However, the researchers factored out olive oil in assessing the health benefits of lycopene.

Uncooked tomatoes had some benefit as well. Although the lycopene is still locked into the fibrous matrix of these tomatoes, uncooked tomatoes are usually eaten as part of a salad that has been dressed with an oil-based dressing or a sandwich of fat-containing meat.

Tomato juice provided no benefits because it is neither cooked nor served with fat or oil.

## Q. Do strawberries contain lycopene?

**A.** Although strawberries proved to be beneficial in this study, they do not contain any lycopene, despite their red color. The benefits of strawberries may be associated with another compound known as ellagic acid—a pigment from a family of compounds called polyphenols.

# Q. Have there been any other studies supporting the protective role of lycopene in prostate cancer?

**A.** Giovannucci conducted two additional studies on the protective role of lycopene in prostate cancer and found the exact same patterns. The more tomato sauce the study subjects consumed, the lower their risk of prostate cancer.

Giovannucci has pointed out that while lycopene is the principal carotenoid found in tomatoes, this food also contains small amounts of beta-carotene and other little known carotenoids, including gamma-carotene, phytoene, phytofluene, and zeta-carotene. It is possible that the entire complex of these carotenoids is better than lycopene alone. However, there is compelling evidence to support the benefits of lycopene by itself.

# Q. How does lycopene work?

**A.** Lycopene is the most powerful antioxidant of all the carotenoids, followed by beta-carotene. As a consequence, lycopene is a very efficient quencher of free radicals and thus reduces the risk of cancer and some age-related diseases. But lycopene, as well as the other carotenoids, has many non-antioxidant functions that seem to influence the behavior of genes. As we learn more about lycopene, we may discover that it activates beneficial genes and deactivates disease-causing genes.

Lycopene seems to predominate in certain organs in the body. For example, the testes and the adrenal glands contain the body's largest stores of lycopene, compared with other organs and glands that contain lycopene, such as the kidneys and the ovaries. When organs retain large amounts of a particular nutrient, it suggests that the nutrient plays an important role in those organs.

## Q. How does lycopene compare with other carotenoids in cancer prevention?

**A.** Though comparative data is very preliminary, laboratory experiments have shown that lycopene was far more effective than beta-carotene and alpha-carotene in inhibiting the growth of cancerous endometrial cells, breast cells, and lung cells. This does not mean lycopene is a cure for cancer. However, such research suggests that lycopene can help prevent some cancers.

# Q. Does lycopene offer any benefits for other prostate problems?

**A.** Some men have used lycopene supplements to reduce benign prostatic hyperplasia, the enlargement of the prostate. Others have used it to treat prostatitis, an inflammation or infection of the prostate. Although lycopene's use for these problems is purely anecdotal and not scientifically proven, it does make sense. Antioxidants such as lycopene tend to have an anti-inflammatory effect, in part because they neutralize the pro-inflammatory effect of free radicals.

# Q. Can lycopene reduce the risk of breast cancer?

**A.** There is tantalizing evidence based on animal research that lycopene can reduce the risk of breast cancer. A team of Japanese researchers has conducted several studies that have found that lycopene can suppress the growth of breast cancer cells in mice in two ways. First, lycopene increases the ratio of protective immune cells known as CD4 cells to CD8 cells, which tend to deactivate the immune response. Second, lycopene also reduces the activity of transforming growth factor alpha—a compound that promotes tumor development.

## Q. Is lycopene of value in any other type of cancer normally associated with women?

**A.** Researchers recently reported that black women who had a high intake of lycopene were one-third less likely to develop cervical dysplasia, or precancerous tissue changes in the cervix. Keep in mind that this study noted an association, not a direct cause and effect.

## Q. Does lycopene have any effect on the risk of lung cancer?

**A.** Animal research has shown that lycopene may reduce the risk of lung cancer. In one study, researchers exposed mice to various cancer-causing chemicals. Some of the mice were given lycopene, while others were not. Those that received the lycopene had fewer cancerous growths, as well as precancerous growths, in the lungs.

# Q. Does lycopene seem to have benefits in any other types of cancer?

A. Research suggests that lycopene may be beneficial in other types of cancer. In a study of eating habits and cancer risk, European researchers found that diets high in uncooked tomatoes were associated with a significant reduction in the risk of stomach cancer and intestinal cancer and showed modest risk reductions in oral, pharynx, and esophageal cancers. Because lycopene is by far the predominant carotenoid in tomatoes, it may be one of the key nutrients influencing the decreased risk of these cancers.

# Q. Does lycopene offer any benefits to the heart?

A. Like most antioxidant nutrients, lycopene has been shown to benefit the heart. A recent study highlighted how high levels of lycopene in the body may reduce the risk of a heart attack. Lycopene and other fat-soluble nutrients are typically stored in the body's adipose, or fat, cells, as well as in the fatty components of other cells. Researchers analyzed the levels of lycopene and other nutrients in the fat tissue of heart attack patients and the fat tissue of healthy subjects from ten European countries. They found that people with the highest lycopene levels were 48-percent less likely to suffer a heart attack.

## Q. How does lycopene reduce the risk of heart disease?

**A.** Because free radicals can injure the heart and blood vessels, these destructive molecules are considered key players in the development of heart disease. They also turn normal LDL cholesterol into oxidized LDL cholesterol, accelerating the development of heart disease. Although cholesterol—particularly the LDL form—is rumored to be harmful to the body, it is actually essential for good health. Among its other functions, LDL cholesterol is the body's medium for transporting fat-soluble micronutrients, such as lycopene, beta-carotene, lutein, and vitamin E, through the bloodstream. Part of what leads to the oxidation of LDL is a lack of antioxidants in the body. So consuming plenty of antioxidants, including lycopene, can lower LDL oxidation, thus reducing the risk of heart disease.

## Q. Has research shown that lycopene can lower cholesterol levels and reduce LDL oxidation?

**A.** Michael Aviram, DSc, of the Technion Israel Institute of Technology, has shown that supplemental lycopene and beta-carotene can partially inhibit the body's production of cholesterol. These substances share some common biochemical pathways in the body, so loading up on these carotenoids essentially leaves less room for cholesterol.

With lower cholesterol levels, a person's antioxidant requirements should decrease, so that a smaller amount of antioxidants may go a longer way in terms of protecting against LDL oxidation. In fact, in other research conducted by Dr. Aviram and his colleagues, lycopene does reduce LDL oxidation. Adding vitamin E further protected LDL against oxidation. In addition, he found that tomato oleoresin—a fatty extract of tomato that contains lycopene and traces of other antioxidants—was better at preventing LDL oxidation than lycopene by itself.

# Q. If I take lycopene in supplemental form, how much should I take?

**A.** A large ripe tomato contains about 4 mg of lycopene. This amount, taken in supplemental form on a daily basis, seems to be very good for health. As studies have shown, greater amounts of tomato foods, particularly tomato sauce, reduce the risk of prostate cancer and other diseases. There does not seem to be any harm from taking higher doses of lycopene, aside from the minor stomach upset that some people experience from taking any type of oral supplement.

# 5.

# Other Carotenoids

Although beta-carotene, lutein, and lycopene are the most common carotenoids, there are actually many other important dietary carotenoids. Among these are alpha-carotene, cryptoxanthin, and astaxanthin. In this chapter, you'll discover some of the ways these carotenoids also contribute to good health.

## Q. What is alpha-carotene?

**A.** Alpha-carotene, which is closely related to beta-carotene, accounts for generally one-third to one-half of the carotenoids found in carrots. Pumpkins are also very rich in alpha-carotene and actually contain slightly more of this carotenoid than they do beta-carotene.

# Q. Does alpha-carotene have any health benefits?

**A.** Like the other carotenoids, most of the benefits attributed to alpha-carotene seem to be related to cancer prevention.

Serious research on alpha-carotene began in Japan in the late 1980s. Michiaki Murakoshi, PhD, and his colleagues at the Kyoto Prefectural University were motivated by the growing body of research on beta-carotene and believed that other carotenoids might also be worth investigating. They discovered that alpha-carotene had powerful anticancer properties in cell-culture experiments. Alpha-carotene delayed or inhibited the growth of various types of cancer cells, including those of the brain, pancreas, and stomach. Of course, cell-culture experiments are far from studies in human beings, but they do indicate the potential benefits of a substance.

# Q. Have there been any human studies with alpha-carotene?

**A.** One of the best human studies involving alpha-carotene examined the eating habits of male smokers in New Jersey. Some of these men had been diagnosed with cancers of the trachea, bronchus, or lung. The diets of these men were compared with the diets of healthy men of comparable age. It was found that those men who consumed a diet low in alpha-carotene had the greatest risk of developing these cancers.

## Q. What is cryptoxanthin?

**A.** Cryptoxanthin is another minor carotenoid, although it is actually composed of two related molecules, beta- and alpha-cryptoxanthin. Cryptoxanthin is found in papayas, peaches, tangerines, and oranges. Cryptoxanthin is second to beta-carotene in terms of the amount of dietary carotenoids that are converted by the body to vitamin A.

Cryptoxanthin, along with other carotenoids and vitamins, forms part of the antioxidant network in human skin. One recent study found that blood levels of cryptoxanthin were lower in women with precancerous cervical dysplasia. And, in a fifteen-year-long study of 15,000 women, researchers noted that women eating foods high in cryptoxanthin had a significantly lower risk of developing cervical cancer.

# Q. What is astaxanthin?

**A.** Astaxanthin is a carotenoid that serves as a common pigment in sea creatures such as salmon and trout. Some carotenoids are even added to the feed of farm-raised fish to enhance their color and sales appeal. Carotenoids also function as antioxidants in the sea creatures they are found in.

In one experiment, researchers in Ireland compared the ability of beta-carotene, lutein, and astaxanthin to protect against UVA light—a specific wavelength of ultraviolet light that can cause sunburn and skin cancer. In this experiment, astaxanthin proved to be more protective than beta-carotene and lutein. In another experiment, researchers noted that astaxanthin could also enhance immune activity.

# Q. Are there any other beneficial carotenoids, and how can I be sure I'm getting enough of them?

**A.** There are many other minor carotenoids that can be found in the diets of people who regularly eat a wide array of fruits and vegetables. Because it is simply not possible to put every beneficial carotenoid into supplemental form, the best way to obtain a diverse selection of carotenoids is by eating a broad assortment of carotenoid-rich foods.

# 6.

# How to Buy and Use Carotenoids

There are many different types of individual carotenoid supplements and mixed carotenoid supplements on the market—enough to sometimes be confusing. As with anything else, it's important to be an educated consumer. In this chapter, you'll find some pointers for buying carotenoid supplements and deciding which products might be the best ones for you to take. Remember, carotenoid supplements can be extremely beneficial, but they are best used to supplement a good diet, not to replace one.

## Q. Which individual carotenoids are sold as supplements?

**A.** Beta-carotene, lutein, and lycopene are sold as individual carotenoid supplements. As discussed in

Chapter 2, beta-carotene comes in two forms, natural and synthetic. The natural form of beta-carotene is superior to the synthetic form. As discussed in Chapter 3, lutein is extracted from marigold flower petals, and is sometimes called marigold extract. It is available in two forms—as free lutein and as lutein ester. And, as discussed in Chapter 4, lycopene is obtained from tomatoes, and is presently available in only one natural form.

These individual carotenoids can enhance relatively specific aspects of health. For instance, beta-carotene can enhance the immune system, increase resistance to sunburn, and increase lung capacity; lutein is essential for vision and may reduce the risk of macular degeneration; and lycopene has been shown to reduce the risk of prostate cancer. If you are at risk of developing any one of these diseases, it may be prudent to take an individual carotenoid supplement.

# Q. What are mixed carotenoids, and are they available as supplements?

**A.** Although some carotenoids are more common than others, nature provides a natural mix, or diversity, of carotenoids in many of the fruits and vegetables available for our consumption. These "mixed" carotenoids tend to have a synergistic or complementary effect that probably contributes to overall health and resistance to disease.

There are a few different forms of mixed carotenoids available in health food stores and pharmacies. They are also available by mail order.

One type of mixed carotenoid supplement contains a large amount of beta-carotene—both the highly desirable 9-cis form and the all-trans form—along with lutein, zeaxanthin, and cryptoxanthin. Another type contains less beta-carotene, but a higher percentage of alpha-carotene. You will also find mixed carotenoids in some multivitamin supplements and multi-antioxidant formulas. Read the labels carefully to find out exactly what these supplements contain.

## Q. Should I buy mixed carotenoid supplements or individual carotenoid supplements?

**A.** A mixed carotenoid supplement more closely approximates the diverse selection of carotenoids that you would find in a diet including many fruits and vegetables, so this type of supplement is probably better for maintaining general health. Individual carotenoid supplements may be better for specific health problems.

Several studies have suggested that mixed carotenoids have superior beneficial effects on the body than individual carotenoids. These beneficial effects included reduced LDL oxidation in smokers; increased white blood cell activity in women with diets lacking carotenoids; and a lower risk of heart attack in some men.

## Q. Why do some labels state carotenoids in milligrams (mg) and others in international units (IU)?

**A.** For many years, beta-carotene was seen only as a precursor to vitamin A, and because vitamin A measurements are always given in international units, beta-carotene was measured in terms of its equivalence to vitamin A. Now that beta-carotene is being recognized for its own antioxidant properties, more companies are listing beta-carotene in terms of milligrams.

Because the body does not convert lutein or lycopene to vitamin A, these nutrients should always appear as milligrams.

## Q. Is there an easy way to convert from milligrams to international units and vice versa?

**A.** If you have a calculator, the conversion process is relatively easy. If a product lists beta-carotene in international units, and you want to know the amount of milligrams, multiply the number of international units by 0.0006. For example, 20,000 IU multiplied by 0.0006 is 12 mg. If a product lists beta-carotene in milligrams, and you want the number of international units, divide the number of milligrams by .0006. For example, 12 mg divided by 0.0006 equals 20,000 IU.

## Q. Will high doses of one particular carotenoid affect other carotenoids?

**A.** The research in this area is a little confusing. There's some evidence that taking high doses of beta-carotene may lower the levels of or flush out the lutein in the body. There is also evidence that taking beta-carotene increases the body's levels of some other carotenoids. In one study conducted over a two-year period, research found that beta-carotene supplements increased the levels of alpha-carotene and lycopene in the body, but the reason for this is not clear. More research needs to be done on how high doses of one carotenoid may or may not affect other carotenoids.

## Q. Are there any side effects from taking carotenoid supplements?

**A.** If you take very high doses of beta-carotene and other carotenoid supplements for many months, you may notice that your hands and feet take on a yellowish color. This is not in any way harmful. However, if the color is undesirable, reduce your carotenoid intake, or stop taking carotenoid supplements for a month or two, and then resume them at a lower dose.

If you smoke more than one pack of cigarettes daily or drink more than one glass of liquor or alcohol daily, you would probably be better off taking your beta-carotene or carotenoids as part of a broader supplement program that includes vitamin C, vitamin E, and selenium.

## Q. What should I do if my doctor advises me against taking carotenoid supplements?

**A.** More and more physicians are taking supplements themselves and are recommending various supplements to patients. Still, there are many skeptical doctors around. If your doctor is one of them, give him or her a copy of this book. You should always demand the best in medical care from your doctor, so it is not unreasonable to ask him or her to look up the scientific references listed at the end of this book before passing judgment on carotenoid supplements.

## Q. Can carotenoids be taken along with vitamins and minerals?

**A.** Nutrients work best as a team, so by all means, carotenoid supplements can and should be taken as part of a comprehensive supplement and health maintenance regimen.

For general health, it's very important to start with a high-potency multivitamin supplement and a separate multimineral supplement. Trying to get all the nutrients in one supplement usually shortchanges something else. (Minerals take up more space in supplements than vitamins do.) To this regimen, consider adding mixed carotenoids; some additional vitamin C to bring your daily total to at least 1,000 mg; some additional vitamin E to bring your daily total up to 400 IU; and for specific problems discussed in this book, consider taking supplements of the appropriate individual carotenoid.

# Conclusion

Carotenoids enrich our lives with color and also with important health benefits. There are many beneficial carotenoids available in nature, and without doubt the best way to obtain a diverse selection of them is by eating a diverse selection of fruits, vegetables, and other plant foods. Unfortunately, most Americans do not eat the often recommended daily servings of fruits and vegetables, so they miss out on this vital group of nutrients.

Beta-carotene, lutein, and lycopene are the predominant carotenoids that can be found in the American diet. Although they are not technically recognized as essential nutrients, these carotenoids are highly beneficial. They have a broad range of effects, including enhancing the immune system and reducing the risks of cancer and heart disease.

Many other beneficial carotenoids are also found in the diet, though they are less common than the others. These carotenoids include alpha-carotene, cryptoxanthin, and astaxanthin.

All of these carotenoids were a basic part of the pre-human and human diets over millions of years of evolution. Many researchers believe that we are dependent on these nutrients for optimal health because of this "coevolution."

Based on the evidence, carotenoids are important nutrients to include in your diet. Ideally, you should get most of these nutrients from the food you eat. But if you don't eat the right foods, taking supplemental carotenoids can help keep your health on track.

# Glossary

**Antioxidants.** Molecules that limit free-radical damage by donating electrons to quench, or neutralize, free radicals.

**Beta-carotene.** One of the principal dietary carotenoids that gives some foods their orange color. It is a precursor to vitamin A.

**Carotenoids.** A family of about 600 chemically related pigments that function as antioxidants. They are found mainly in fruits, vegetables, and plant greens.

**Cholesterol.** A fatty substance used by the body to build cell walls and produce necessary chemicals. High blood levels of cholesterol have been associated with an increased risk of cardiovascular disease.

**Deoxyribonucleic acid (DNA).** The molecule that forms the basis of genetics, and provides cells with instructions on how to behave. When DNA becomes mutated, or damaged, it increases the risk of degenerative diseases, such as cancer.

**Free radical.** An unpaired electron, produced by the body or pollutants, that tries to stabilize by stealing an electron from another molecule. Unless quenched, free radicals can damage DNA, fats, and proteins; and in doing so, contribute to the aging process and disease.

**Lutein.** One of the principal dietary carotenoids that gives some foods their yellow color.

**Lycopene.** One of the principal dietary carotenoids that gives foods such as tomatoes their red color.

**Provitamin A.** A carotenoid, such as beta-carotene or cryptoxanthin, that the body converts to vitamin A.

**Vitamin A.** A dietary nutrient that is essential for vision.

**Xanthophyll.** A subcategory of carotenoids that generally includes yellowish pigments, such as lutein and zeaxanthin.

**Zeaxanthin.** A carotenoid that is found along with lutein in macular pigment.

# References

Albanes D, Heinonen OP, Taylor PR, et al., "Alpha-tocopherol and beta-carotene supplements and lung cancer incidence in the Alpha-Tocopherol, Beta-Carotene Cancer Prevention study: effects of baseline characteristics and study compliance," *Journal of the National Cancer Institute* 88 (1996):1560–1570.

The Alpha-Tocopherol, Beta-Carotene Cancer Prevention Study Group, "The effect of vitamin E and beta carotene on the incidence of lung cancer and other cancers in male smokers," *New England Journal of Medicine* 330 (1994):1029–1035.

Ben-Amotz A, Levy Y, "Bioavailability of a natural isomer mixture compared with synthetic all-trans beta-carotene in human serum," *American Journal of Clinical Nutrition* 63 (1996):729–734.

Bone RA, Landrum JT, Friedes LM, Gomez CM, Kilburn MD, Menendez E, et al., "Distribution of lutein and zeaxanthin stereoisomers in the human retina," *Experimental Eye Research* 64 (1997):211–218.

Carotenoid Research Interactive Group, "Beta-carotene and the carotenoids: beyond the intervention trials," *Nutrition Reviews* 56 (1996):185–186.

Challem JJ, "Re: Risk factors for lung cancer and for intervention effects in CARET, the Beta-carotene and Retinol Efficacy Trial," *Journal of the National Cancer Institute* 89 (1997):325.

Challem JJ, "Beta-carotene and other carotenoids: promises, failures, and a new vision," *Journal of Orthomolecular Medicine* 12 (1997):11–19.

Chopra M and Thurnham DI, "Effect of lutein on oxidation of low-density lipoproteins (LDL) in vitro," *Proceedings of the Nutrition Society* 53 (1994): 1993, #18A.

Chuwers P, Barnhart S, Blanc P, et al., "The protective effect of B-carotene and retinol on ventilatory function in an asbestos-exposed cohort," *American Journal of Respiratory and Critical Care Medicine* 155 (1997):1066–1071.

Clinton SK, "Lycopene: chemistry, biology, and implications for human health and disease," *Nutrition Reviews* 56 (1998):35–51.

Furhman B, Ben-Yaish L, Attias J, et al., "Tomato lycopene and beta-carotene inhibit low density lipoprotein oxidation and this effect depends on the lipoprotein vitamin E content," *Nutrition Metabolism and Cardiovascular Diseases* 7 (1997):433–443.

Garewal HS, et al., "Emerging role of beta-carotene and antioxidant nutrients in prevention of oral cancer," *Archives of Otolaryngology* 121 (1995):141–144.

Gollnick HPM, Hopfenmüller, Hemmes C, "Systemic beta carotene plus topical UV-sunscreen are an optimal protection against harmful effects of natural UV-sunlight: results of the Berline-Eilath study," *European Journal of Dermatology* 6 (1996):200–205.

Giovannucci E, Ascherio A, Rimm EB, et al., "Intake of carotenoids and retinol in relation to risk of prostate cancer," *Journal of the National Cancer Institute* 87 (1995):1767–1776.

Hammond Jr BR, Fuld K, and Curran-Celentano J, "Macular pigment in monozygotic twins," *Investigative Ophthalmology and Visual Science* 36 (1995): 2431–2441.

Handelman GJ, "Carotenoids as scavengers of active oxygen species." *In Handbook of Antioxidants,* Cadenas E and Packer L, eds: Marcel Dekker, New York, 1996.

Hennekens CH, Buring JE, Manson JE, et al., "Lack of effect of long-term supplementation with beta-carotene on the incidence of malignant neoplasms and cardiovascular disease," *New England Journal of Medicine* 334 (1996):1145–1149.

Howard AN, Williams NR, Palmer CR, Cambou JP, Evans AE, Foote JW, et al., "Do hydroxy-carotenoids prevent coronary heart disease? A comparison between Belfast and Toulouse," *International Journal of Vitamin and Nutrition Research* 66 (1996):113–118.

Hughes DA, Wright AJA, Finglas PM, et al., "The effect of B-carotene supplementation on the immune function of blood monocytes from healthy male nonsmokers," *Journal of Laboratory and Clinical Medicine* 129 (1997):309–317.

Kazi N, Radvany R, Oldham T, et al., "Immuno-modulatory effect of B-carotene on T lymphocyte subsets in patients with resected colonic polyps and cancer," *Nutrition and Cancer* 28 (1997):140–145.

Khachik F, Beecher GR, and Smith JC, "Lutein, lycopene, and their oxidative metabolites in chemoprevention of cancer," *Journal of Cellular Biology* 22 (1995):236–246.

Kohlmeier L, Kark JD, Gomez-Garcia B, et al., "Lycopene and myocardial infarction risk in the EURAMIC study," *American Journal of Epidemiology* 146 (1997):618–626.

Kramer TR and Burri BJ, "Modulated mitogenic proliferative responsiveness of lymphocytes in wholeblood cultures after a low-carotene diet and mixed-carotenoid supplementation in women," *American Journal of Clinical Nutrition* 65 (1997):871–875.

Landrum JT, Bone RA, Joa H, Kilbourn MD, Moore LL, and Sprague KE, "A one year study of the macular pigment: the effect of 140 days of a lutein supplement," *Experimental Eye Research* 65 (1997):57–62.

Lin Y, Burri BJ, Neidlinger TR, "Estimating the concentration of b-carotene required for maximal protection of low-density lipoproteins in women," *American Journal of Clinical Nutrition* 67 (1998):837–845.

Morris DL, et al., "Serum carotenoids and coronary heart disease. The Lipid Research Clinics Coronary Primary Prevention Trial and Follow-up Study," *Journal of the American Medical Association* 272 (1994): 1439–1441.

Morris DL, Kritchevsky SB, Davis CE, "Serum carotenoids and coronary heart disease. The Lipid Research Clinics Coronary Primary Prevention Trial and Follow-up Study," *Journal of the American Medical Association* 272 (1994):1439–1441

Murad H and Challem J, "Free radicals and antioxidants in dermatology," *Cosmetic Dermatology* 10 (1994):39–43.

Murakoshi M, et al., "Potent preventive action of alpha-carotene against carcinogenesis: Spontaneous liver carcinogenesis and promoting stage of lung and skin carcinogenesis in mice are suppressed more effectively by alpha-carotene than by beta-carotene," *Cancer Research* 52 (1992):6583–6587.

Nagasawa H, Mitamura T, Sakamoto S, et al., "Effects of lycopene on spontaneous mammary tumour development in SHN virgin mice," *Anticancer Research* 15 (1995): 1173–1178.

Omenn GS, Goodman GE, Thornquist MD, et al., "Effects of a combination of beta carotene and vitamin A on lung cancer and cardiovascular disease," *New England Journal of Medicine* 334 (1996): 1150–1155.

Omenn GS, Goodman GE, Thornquist MD, et al., "Risk factors for lung cancer and for intervention effects in CARET, the beta-carotene and retinol efficacy trial," *Journal of the National Cancer Institute* 88 (1996):1550–1559.

Park JS, Chew BP, Wong TS, "Dietary lutein from marigold extract inhibits mammary tumor development in BALB/c mice," *Journal of Nutrition* 128 (1998):1650–1656.

Seddon JM, Ajani UA, Sperduto RD, Hiller R, Blair N, Burton TC, et al., "Dietary carotenoids, vitamins A, C, and E, and advanced age-related macular degeneration," *Journal of the American Medical Association* 272 (1994):1413–1420.

Street DA, et al., "Serum antioxidants and myocardial infarction. Are low levels of carotenoids and alpha-tocopherol risk factors for myocardial infarction?" *Circulation* 90 (1994):1154–1161.

Umegaki K, et al., "Beta-carotene prevents x-ray induction of micronuclei in human lymphocytes," *American Journal of Clinical Nutrition* 59 (1994): 409–412.

Zhou JR, Gugger ET, Erdman JW Jr, "The crystalline form of carotenes and the food matrix in carrot root decrease the relative bioavailability of beta- and alpha-carotene in the ferret model," *Journal of the American College of Nutrition* 15 (1996):84–91.

Ziegler RG, Subar AF, Craft NE, et al., "Does beta-carotene explain why reduced cancer risk is associated with vegetable and fruit intake?" *Cancer Research* 52 (1992):2060–2066.

# Suggested Readings

Challem J, *All About Vitamins*. Garden City Park, New York: Avery Publishing Group, 1998.

Challem J and Smith MD, *All About Vitamin E*. Garden City Park, New York: Avery Publishing Group, 1999.

Lieberman S and Bruning N, *The Real Vitamin and Mineral Book*. Garden City Park, New York: Avery Publishing Group, 1997.

# Index